DOCTOR, DOCTOR

DOCTOR DOCTOR

Life Lessons of a Veterinarian
Turned Physician

DR. JOANNE HOLLAND

WITH TOM ALESIA

COUNCIL TRAIL PRESS
Arlington Heights, Illinois

Published by
Council Trail Press
Arlington Heights, Illinois

Printed in the United States of America

Designed by Sara DeHaan

ISBN (paper) 979-8-218-57378-2
ISBN (ebook) 979-8-218-57377-5.

To Jennifer and Anna,
with my apologies

Dr. Joanne Holland

To Susan, Mark and Lincoln

Tom Alesia

Contents

Foreword

In deep winter January 1994, my wife and I bought a puppy, the last West Highland White Terrier (or, simply, Westie) available at a generic, franchise pet store in Madison, Wisconsin. The tiny puffball—who we named Lincoln, because we had moved to Madison from Abraham Lincoln's longtime home of Springfield, Illinois—quickly needed a checkup. To meet our day-time work schedules, the only option was a veterinarian with evening hours.

On the night of our appointment, Lincoln shook as the temperatures dipped like a dropped bowling ball. We also knew that the generic, franchise pet store was a poor place for puppies.

When we entered the Arboretum Animal Clinic, with its weathered exterior in a former small home, there was no receptionist or vet tech. Instead, the one-woman clinic was Dr. Joanne Holland's workplace. After quick pleasantries, Holland took the shivering Lincoln and wrapped him in a blanket as tightly as foil on an uneaten chicken leg. Then she sat in a chair and held him near her heat vent.

Holland heard us describe our fears, especially that we supported a place far more interested in profit over its pets' well-being. For several minutes, she listened to our story; two young adults over their heads with a puppy needing care.

When she spoke, Holland acknowledged our pet-store purchase guilt.

"What's done is done," she said. "But you saved him."

Then she examined Lincoln as we shifted from the office's lobby—covered with polaroids and other pictures of hundreds of pet patients—to the work area. We were the only people at the clinic and the clock neared her closing time, but she acted as if she had all the time in the world. She explained to two puppy novices how we would strengthen Lincoln and assured us that he would become healthier in a few weeks.

Holland was Lincoln's vet for the next six years— right up until Holland shocked us with news: She had been in medical school throughout those years. The veteran veterinarian was about to stop her practice to begin her residency on the West Coast.

At the time, I was a features writer for the Wisconsin State Journal in Madison. Holland's story about her impending med school graduation earned front-page attention. Years later, I formed a website with some of my favorite stories that I had written. Holland's profile was included, and others who visited the website asked me: What happened to her?

A quick Google search in 2021 uncovered her as a 17-year doctor—still practicing!—in a remote city called Drain in Oregon.

In my original newspaper story, I asked a spokesperson at the University of Wisconsin Medical School about Holland's stunning accomplishment to graduate despite so many obstacles: age, single motherhood, life-threatening illnesses, dyslexia, a school/work combination and financial strain.

"Any *one* of those (situations)," the spokesperson said, "has kept individuals out in the past."

Out of the blue, I called Holland's medical clinic in Drain. She answered the phone.

I told her that I wanted to finish her incredible story—this time, as a book.

She hesitated but agreed. We spent countless hours doing interviews.

"Will anyone," she asked, "believe this?"

Dr. Joanne Holland
Timeline

March 18, 1945: Born in Flint, Mich.

June 1963: Graduated Nicolet High School, Glendale, Wisc., struggling with undiagnosed dyslexia.

Summer 1963: After being accepted by Iowa State University, she received a postcard from the school: "We do not accept women in the school of veterinary medicine." Iowa State officials reversed their stance when Holland and her mother complained vehemently in person.

Late 1966 and early 1967: Traveled to Saigon with a tourist visa to meet her soldier boyfriend and to see Vietnam for herself during the war.

May 1969: Became one of the first women to graduate from the Iowa State University School of Veterinary Medicine after facing sexism throughout her six years there.

1971: Moved to Fairbanks, Alaska, with her first husband, Peter, who struggled with PTSD after the Vietnam War and hoped that moving to a remote area would help him mentally.

Winter 1974-1975: Lived in a cabin in the Alaskan bush, where she treated animals for a meager income.

1975: Moved to Whitehorse in Canada's Yukon Territory and opened the only veterinary clinic within a 500-mile radius.

1979: Alone, raised two daughters, including one with autism.

1982: Formed a one-person veterinary clinic in Madison, Wisconsin.

1992-1993: While running her veterinary clinic, she studied from 4-6 a.m. daily for the medical school entrance exam.

July/August 1994: Accepted to University of Wisconsin-Madison School of Medicine. Then took classes while keeping her veterinary practice going part time for almost six years.

Dr. Joanne Holland Timeline

1998: Needed emergency, life-saving surgery to remove a "mouse-sized" tumor inside her heart.

1999: Suffered a burst appendix.

January 2000: Graduated from medical school.

August 2000: Began a residency for rural medicine in Oregon.

Early 2004: Opened a one-person medical clinic in Drain, Oregon, at age 60.

Present: Practices medicine on a part-time basis in rural Oregon.

Things Turn Out the Way
They Are Supposed To

The full moon looks down upon
the empty street with the same face
it would have if the street were full.
My face is illuminated from this morning walk.
The snow holds the moon's blue light under my feet.
All is gone when the clouds move before the moon.

—JOANNE HOLLAND,
February 1989

CHAPTER ONE

Veterinarian to Medical School

Be a risk taker—
but not a silly risk taker-type,
or one who likes risks for the sake of risks.
Do it for intellectual reasons.

In 1991, one of my canine patients, a husky and German shepherd mix, gave me Lyme disease. I got it from exposure: blood on blood. I turned to put the dog's blood in a container, and the dog pulled back. My hand was on the wrong side of the hole that I just poked, and blood poured out onto a cat scratch that had happened earlier that day. Like many veterinarians, I tended to be blasé about this kind of thing, especially after 22 years in practice in urban Wisconsin, frontier Alaska, the Yukon Territory, and back to Wisconsin. After that, I was an advocate of covering up your damn wounds. Don't be freaking brave.

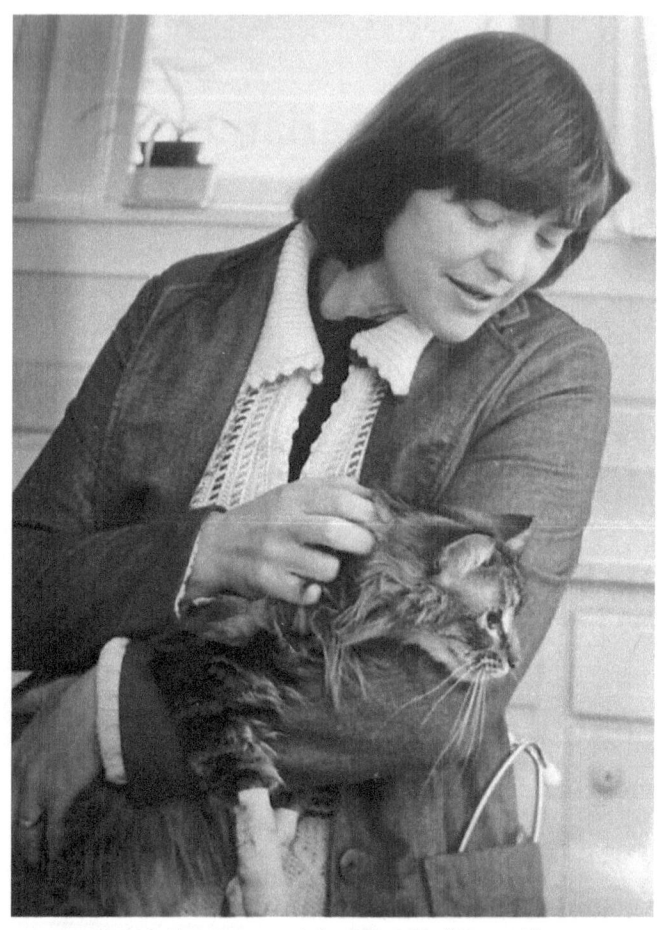

Dr. Holland at work in the veterinary office

When I was infected, I wiped off the blood because veterinarians are tough. A week later, I had a joint problem and a fever. I spent the next year treating my Lyme disease. I couldn't prepare for Christmas. My two daughters put the Christmas tree up. We brought in pizzas, something I'd never done before. At work, I placed stools throughout my one-person vet clinic in Madison, Wisconsin, so I could sit and take my antibiotics. I was exhausted. Oh, my gosh.

This gave me time to think. And that meant exploring life's possibilities and potential opportunities.

At the time, I was moving into research, but I loved practicing medicine so much more. I started thinking about doing *human* medicine.

I was 45 years old and an accomplished veterinarian. The switch to medical school plus the rigorous, post-graduate residency would take at least six or seven years. I helped pets for years. Now I started thinking about caring for pet owners—and all people, especially rural ones with few healthcare choices.

It seemed perfectly logical in a weird way. I was taking classes in animal therapy; I had been taking classes in psychology. I was interested in doing behavioral work. If I got a PhD in psychology and animal behavioral work, I would make less money than I do as a vet. Why would I do that? So, I thought, maybe I should apply to medical school.

It did not take long to decide that I really wanted this. I'm a risk taker—but not a silly risk taker-type. Not one of these people who likes risks for the sake of risks. In this case, it was intellectual.

I kept seeing all these pet owners that I knew who were relatively poor and getting dreadful healthcare, but their dogs were doing fine. Your veterinary care is better than your human care? Give me a break!

Of course, I wasn't sure if I could get accepted to med school.

I didn't apply until early 1994, when I was 49 years old. At best, I could finish med school and its residency when I was 55 or 56. This would still make me one of the oldest med school grads ever—and one of the oldest doctors who planned to practice medicine for nearly 20 years.

My age was just one factor to consider. I was an overworked single mother—twice divorced, both terrible situations—with two teenage daughters, including one with autism.

Oh, and I'm dyslexic!

Which means I would have to get through med

school with a learning disorder that affects reading and writing.

For two years, during my free time, I studied for the MCATs (Medical College Admissions Test). I got up at 4 a.m. and studied for two hours then got breakfast ready.

My application essay emphasized how members of my family often lived long lives. I told almost nobody that I applied. I didn't tell my elderly parents because I didn't know if I'd get in. My daughters knew what I was studying for; they knew I wanted to be a medical doctor. I applied only at the University of Wisconsin-Madison. I couldn't go elsewhere because of my family. Medical schools publish statistics about their class MCAT scores, demographics, experiences and so on. I compared myself to that, and I knew I had a slim chance.

Sure enough, I was put on the waitlist. Other applicants applied at lots of different places, and I learned I was about number 50 on the waitlist. I needed a lot of other applicants to pick other schools—and, remarkably, that happened.

By June 1994, two months before school started, an admissions worker called me with some good news.

"Joanne, you're within 10 spots now," she said. "You're almost certain to get in."

I didn't have time to celebrate, although I was thrilled, positively thrilled, and anxious. I started to taper off my full-time vet clinic, but that took most of my first year of med school. I eventually saw animals for two hours in evenings and on Saturdays. In a humorous moment, I joined AARP before med school started.

My life had two new goals: to become a doctor and to help a rural community—any small town—by easing patients' health insurance snarls.

I am now about to turn 79 years old and still practicing in tiny Drain, Oregon. My life has expanded from a suburban Milwaukee childhood when I was painfully shy and dubbed an underachieving student due to my undiagnosed dyslexia. I was saved by animals; we always bonded. Then I graduated from an absurdly sexist veterinary college, where ridicule toward female students was common.

My personal life was a similar struggle. I was never good at picking soulmates. I joined my first husband, suffering severely from PTSD after fighting in Vietnam, who wanted to live in Alaska. As a result, I spent the 1970s working in frigid Fairbanks then ran my own one-person practice in Whitehorse, a city in Canada's isolated Yukon Territory.

I returned to Wisconsin and, after spending two years in a vet practice in rural Monroe, opened the Arboretum Animal Clinic in Madison. That allowed me enough flexibility to help my youngest daughter, Anna, through autism's maze.

Then I got Lyme disease, and I ended up in med school a few years later. My classmates were so young. Then tragedy struck again. And again. In 1998, I made it through classes—after the removal of a life-threatening tumor, a myxoma the size of a mouse, in my heart.

Just a year after heart surgery, I went to the Emergency Room with stomach pains. I told the ER doctor that I had appendicitis. Later, the doctor poked around, and I didn't make the usual distress sounds of someone with that condition. I said I couldn't talk, except to say that I was dealing with the excruciating pain. So, the doctor told me to wait for a while and he would check back. A short time later, my appendix burst. That led to complex surgery and caused part of my colon to be removed.

Less than a year after that, I graduated med school.

I'm headstrong.

I'm a survivor.

I'm proud to have practiced medicine in Drain, Oregon, for almost 20 years.

Nothing came easily.

Not one thing.

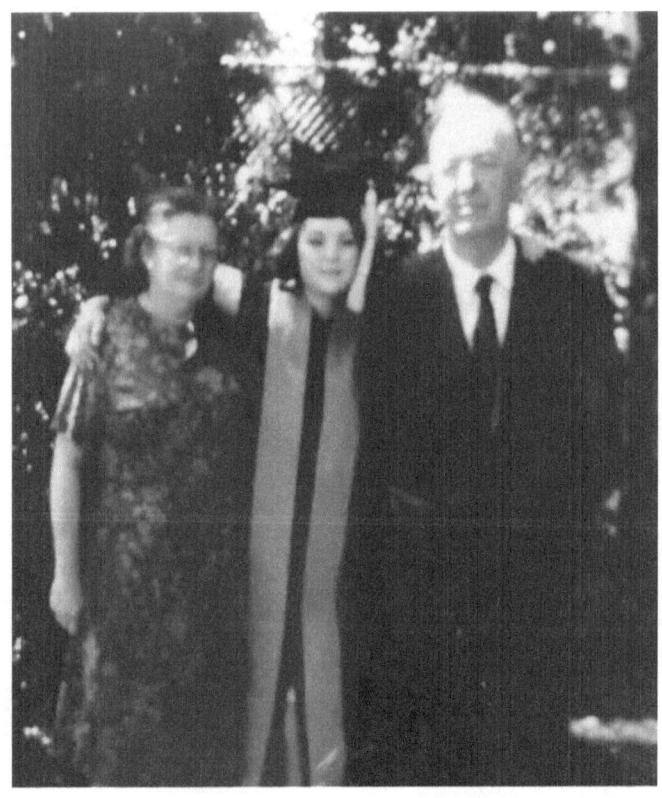

Holland with her parents at Iowa State
Vet School Graduation in 1969.

CHAPTER TWO

Morphine Trickery

Don't let the creeps stop you.

During my senior year of high school, after I applied for the pre-vet program, Iowa State University officials sent me a postcard. It said: "We do not accept women in the school of veterinary medicine. Please reply with your second choice for career."

My mother was livid. The school had already accepted me almost immediately, so this message seemed bizarre. And, at that time, you could, if you really stuck to it, take enough credits and graduate from vet school in six years.

During spring break, my mom and I went to Iowa State in Ames with the postcard in hand. She went to the dean of the veterinary school and said, "What is this?"

He mumbled, "What?" The man blushed. "Oh, well, uh, that's not really true."

They were embarrassed because they were breaking the law. I mean, you can't keep women out of the vet school! Was the postcard an accident? Absolutely not. I learned quickly, once I started the program, that they were not kind to women. There were five women in the class, up from two the year before, and about 70 men.

To change clothes, all five of us used the janitor's closet. Women wore nylons and a frock. We had to go to the barns, and we had to put on our overalls—with nylons—where animals were kicking around. It was crazy.

As a freshman and sophomore, I was a pre-vet student, and I did well. I felt more motivated because of the verbal abuse toward women at that time.

I already was incredibly involved with the nuts and bolts of animal care. I had been out on the farm, working with pigs and helping with pigs being born. I had a lot of experience. It's all I wanted to do. I had to memorize a lot of information, but that was no problem.

Sexism was rampant at Iowa State in the mid and late 1960s. Imagine being someplace where you have 70-some compatriots, and none of them will talk to you. Not one. If they worked on a project with you, they didn't say a word. I was an outcast. I smoked at the time, and when I went out for a smoke, there would be eight guys out there making dirty jokes and turning their backs on me.

At Iowa State University, there was the Junior

Veterinarian Medicine Association. To join, you had to go to meetings and sign in. One of the students, nearing his graduation, would make jokes about some of the doctors and how they held the dogs.

Far worse, other students made jokes about the women—sometimes specifying which woman by name. So, I would go to the meeting, all dressed up, surrounded by everyone, and they'd make obscene jokes about one of the women in your class and everyone laughed. No one was ashamed.

Most women quit going to the Junior Veterinary Medicine Association meetings. I wrote a letter of complaint to the school administrators, but no one apologized. I was too shy to go public about this stuff. I told the people who were heading that department, and they said it would change. So, I went back to the meetings, but nothing much changed.

Since then, I've worked and lived in rural areas. In some rural areas, they make obscene jokes—or jokes in which you make obscene innuendo about a female member or a teenage girl that they know. It's a common thing in rural areas. It's not uncommon in some families: people say, "You know so and so," then tell a joke about her. Even at

Christmas dinner. I hate it. I've seen it. My tawdry grand-father-in-law did it. What they were doing at Iowa State wasn't uncommon enough for them to feel uncomfortable about it.

Iowa wanted to keep high achieving veterinarians in Iowa. They wanted you in veterinary school, especially if you were from a rural area. For veterinary medicine there were six applicants for every space. About half the class was poor, rural Iowans with spotty educations. They were good enough students, but if Shakespeare was mentioned, they'd say, "Yeah, *that's* the guy" and ridicule him. They were comfortable with that. The women weren't. We stared straight ahead. I never thought about leaving Iowa State, though. I was too stubborn. Don't tell me I can't do this.

One of the five girls that I started with moved to California. Another dropped out. Only three graduated. One was a lesbian; the other one was blowsy and sweet, a western kind of girl; she would make jokes back at them. But they changed her name in the graduating class picture to "Buster Cherry."

I stayed. Why let these creeps stop me? I didn't date any of them. There wasn't a prayer, though, that I would get my veterinary license in Iowa. Instead, I got my degree and went to work in Milwaukee.

In summer 1969 after graduation, I worked with Dr. Nicholson at the Small Animal Hospital in Milwaukee. He was right across the street from my dad's job at the city's original General Motors plant, which he helped choose the location of when he worked there.

My dad went to Dr. Nicholson and said, "By the way, my kid's graduating. Are you going to take her in for an internship?" It worked. So, I was an intern then he offered me a full-time job and I took it. We were quite different. He was a right-wing man with the John Birch Society.

I looked like a high school student, even at age 24. I spent one year there on Brady Street in Milwaukee. It was wild down there. I had an apartment right down the street.

At the animal hospital, someone broke in looking for drugs. It happened twice! After the first time, Dr. Nicholson was mad. "Those hippies!" he shouted.

After the first theft, I said, "Let's fix it in case it ever happens again." I put something called "apomorphine" in an obvious place. "Apomorphine" is not morphine. It will make you vomit. It's used to clear stomachs and get bad things out.

The second time we were robbed the thieves took *that*.

CHAPTER THREE

I Went to Vietnam During the War

Anyone who speaks three languages sounds good.

Immediately after graduating from Iowa State vet school, I got married. I had an obligatory trip to Europe at the end of sophomore year as a pre-vet. I had a roommate. I was not very social in the dorms. I found an apartment. My roommate and I went to the Netherlands, and I ran into this guy. He was intriguing. He was American; a military guy who was between stints. He dropped out of the military then he was going to start back up again. He wanted to go back to Germany where he was born. We met at the student hostel in Amsterdam.

His name was Peter Schmidt. When he went back to the military, he was in Vietnam, and he wrote to me. At that time, I was ignorant about this whole "loving thing." I wasn't planning on getting married. But, about the time that I graduated veterinary school in 1969, we were married. I was a Catholic at the time, and I had those mores, and I thought I was going to help someone out. It was an error. Three years later, we were divorced.

We lived in Milwaukee. He was a laborer; I worked as a veterinarian. He had PTSD from the war. He was born in Germany, but his mother had brought him over here quite young. He was three years older than me. It was romantic. He spoke three languages. But he wasn't nice. He wasn't abusive, but he was dangerous, and I was worried about him. We'd go out to eat and he'd say, "I could kill that waitress."

When he went to Vietnam, I don't think he thought I was going to respond to his letters. He spent three years in Vietnam. It was awful fighting. He would write back and say how many people had been killed and how he hated his commander. I would try to support him. He wasn't bad looking. Anyone who spoke more than one language was good to me. He wasn't stupid, but he wasn't educated. Vietnam ruined his life.

And I went there.

To Vietnam.

During the war.

I went to Vietnam for a couple of weeks in late 1966 and early 1967. It was a complex thing. Between 1963 and 1969, there was a huge cultural change in teenagers and young adults regarding behavior and their ideas. Iowa was a very conservative state, but a few people were anti-war in 1963. By 1965, there were more of them. It was the start of the flower child period: hair was down to your ass. We wore pattern stockings, short skirts, and hair all teased.

I wanted to see Peter, who was my boyfriend at the time, but contact was slim. We wrote letters, and he called a few times; I heard gunshots in the background. That was uncomfortable. I tried to find out what was going on with the war, but it was difficult, particularly in Ames, Iowa. Most people were very pro-war. Then there were others who shouted about murderers and showed pictures of people with melting faces, saying, "This is how evil we are."

We were either saving the world for democracy or we were evil murderers. I wanted to find out what was really happening.

I knew a guy who was surveying Iowa State students about the war since we couldn't go there.

"What do you mean you can't go to Vietnam?" I said. "I'll bet you can go."

He said, "You can't."

I said, "I bet you can."

I got a passport and called a travel agency and, sure enough, I could buy a ticket! The travel agent told me I needed government permission through a visa. So, I wrote a letter to some bureaucrat asking how to get a visa to go to Vietnam. It came back and one of the ways was to list "tourist." I showed this to the travel agent, and I got a visa. The travel agent didn't believe it would work. He said, "You'll never get in."

I bought a ticket to Vietnam for two weeks during school's Christmas break in late 1966 and early 1967. It wasn't very expensive.

I contacted Peter and said, "I'm coming to Saigon. Do you think you can see me?"

My friend was more adventurous than me; she was a pre-med student named Sue Anderson. She said, "That's a great idea. I'm going with you." And so, we went. It was a complex place to be. We stayed one night at an expensive hotel in Saigon, but then I looked around for a cheap place and found it. After we moved in, I realized it was a brothel. We could lock the door, but it wasn't strong.

The South Vietnamese thought we were nuts, but they were very nice. This was just before the Tet Offensive when the North Vietnamese and Vietcong mounted a major attack.

My boyfriend, Peter, snuck away, went AWOL and came to Saigon to stay with me for five days. We would go and eat breakfast at this other hotel and hang out and talk. We went to some of the bars. I imagine people thought we were dipshit crazy kids. Then Peter went back to his troop without any trouble.

Sue and I traveled around Saigon. We got Vietnamese dresses. When we were in the brothel hotel, you could go on the roof and watch the war. You could see it like fireworks. It was a good distance away. People started out friendly, but I grew uncomfortable. The war was so close.

During the day, we shopped for trinkets, but I began to feel people were looking at us oddly. I remember cleaning up a park and throwing the garbage into a waste-basket. When I returned there, somebody had taken all the stuff and carefully put it right back down all over the ground. I took this as a sign that we weren't wanted.

I went to the airport and got my ticket changed to come home a day or two early. My friend got a job, so she stayed in Saigon. She told her employer that she could take shorthand even though she couldn't. But she could take notes quickly and type, so she got a job doing that for a multinational corporation.

We learned there that we couldn't discover what was happening in Vietnam—even being there. The people who knew what was going on—on both sides—weren't telling anybody. Both sides were burning things down. That's what I discovered: There was no truth to what was happening. Later, I learned how it evolved. At the time, it was a very complex situation. They interpreted it as neocolonialism, and we interpreted it as a fight against communists.

In Saigon, I got on a plane and landed back in Des Moines about 24 hours before the start of the Tet Offensive. My friend had already moved to an apartment where the corporation encouraged her to move.

A lot of people were trying to get out of Saigon at that time. It was a poorly kept secret that the Tet Offensive was coming—at least among the Vietnamese. The airport was really crowded, and there were long lines. The entire airport was guarded by American military police. This nice young man got me out of line and took me up and walked me out to the plane. I was ushered through. I later wrote him a letter of thanks. I got a letter back that he had died during the Tet Offensive.

Sue wrote to me. She had to dodge bullets across the road to hide in a building to get home on some days. She stayed until the spring. She worked there for about six months.

That was the "Cloud of War." There were missionaries on the plane to Saigon with goals that were completely unachievable. The Vietnamese I met were nice. But we were clueless.

Still, I had an extraordinary experience in Vietnam. We talked to Vietnamese people and the people at the Grand Hotel. Because we were cute "kids," people would buy us beers. We'd sit down and a couple of guys would come over. Contractors were working for money. Vietnamese street kids ran around, trying to get people to buy them something.

It was a country with a lot of social inequities. The country had no desire to be friends with Americans; they kept their distance. It reconfirmed the theory that we were colonizers.

As I look back on that odd and potentially dangerous trip, I think for me it was a way to rebel against the relatively staid requirements of my veterinary school, where we were all supposed to be just so nice from nine to five every day. I mean, I told my parents I was going on a ski trip. My mother knew the truth, I think.

CHAPTER FOUR

In Alaska to Save
My Husband

*There are easier ways
to discover that you need only the basics in life
than living in a cabin in the Alaskan bush.*

I was about to graduate from veterinary school when Peter returned from Vietnam, and we decided to get married. My father almost didn't go to the wedding. He thought Peter was not up to par. I was not very competent at "people" things. I was good at reading animals and not good at reading people. What did I know about relationships?

We married in Ames, Iowa, where Iowa State University is located. There were a lot of alternative lifestyles going on in 1969. We found some little, off-brand Protestant guy who was willing to marry us in a week. I was married in a mini skirt. We got married in a wab, or the area immediately surrounding a sundial, as in Lewis Carroll's "Jabberwocky."

My dad was happy that I'd graduated and hosted a big dinner for me at a park and had everyone come up from his tiny hometown of Bradford, Illinois. My parents were very proud that I graduated from veterinary school. My parents were always civil and didn't say what they thought, but they tolerated my boyfriend, who became my husband.

I was also truly incompetent at human interactions. I remembered my dreams quite vividly, but there were no human beings in my dreams until I was in my 40s. I remembered places and animals. (Two decades later, I had a dream with the streets full of people and, from then on, I was much better with people. Unusual, I know.)

Before Peter came home from Vietnam, the military offered soldiers two choices: Go to Camp Pendleton in California to spend three weeks decompressing and getting ready for life at home again; or get a plane ticket straight home. Peter, like everyone else, chose the ticket home. He couldn't wait to get home.

Because most of those soldiers chose to come directly home meant they wouldn't have any care at all for the diseases they'd acquired while they were in Vietnam. When Peter arrived in Milwaukee from Vietnam, he was only 24 hours removed from artillery fire. He looked like someone had shot him between the eyes. This was the beginning of a really difficult time.

I didn't know anything about depression. I didn't know anything about PTSD. I didn't know how human beings react to war. My husband, Peter, bless his heart, was distinctly troubled. He was miserable. He felt if he could find the right place, he would be better. I thought, "Well, if he would be happy somewhere else …" My family was in Milwaukee, so I figured he wanted us to start somewhere on our own. I didn't realize that it wouldn't matter where we were; he was going to be unhappy.

So, we went to Alaska.

It was the Last Frontier.

In 1971, we drove an old Jeep from Milwaukee to Fairbanks. We brought an extra tire along. And we needed it.

Fairbanks was sprawling and very rural. A lot of mosquitoes. We didn't have much money.

In the time since he had been back in the United States, Peter would wake up in the middle of the night screaming, but while we were traveling that stopped. It was an adventure living there. I got a job as a lab tech at the University of Alaska-Fairbanks. I worked in the experimental laboratory for forestry, mostly measuring samples. It took me a year to study and pass the veterinary boards to be a licensed vet in Alaska. I was still better able to deal with animals than with people.

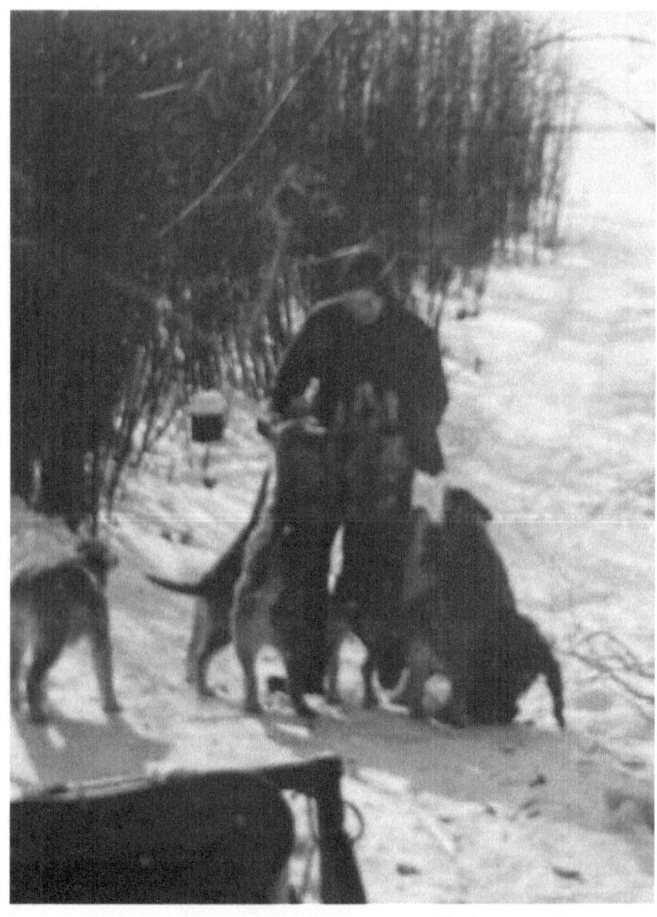

Holland greeted by dogs on an Alaskan path.

I ended up working with a veterinarian who had been up there forever: Dr. Beckley. But when I was in Anchorage to take the state's veterinary exam, we had an odd situation. All the veterinarians gathered there, and they knew each other. After the exam, people who took the test came back to the hotel where we were all staying, and everyone went for drinks. As it got late, suddenly, there were four drinks in front of me and there was the head of the exam board next to me. It was sexual harassment. You'd lose your license now. The extra drinks had been sent by other veterinarians suggesting, "Hey, have a try at her, Dr. Beckley." At me!

But when he hired me, I didn't have a choice but to work for him. I wanted to have a job, and I couldn't have a clinic on my own. He never hit on me again—I think that line had been drawn clearly—and I did learn a lot from him.

He was 50 when I met him in 1971. When he'd come to Alaska originally, he was one of the only veterinarians. He was a crotchety, old guy. When I was interviewed for the job, I heard him call someone and shout, "This is 'Beck.' You owe me $50. I want you to pay it!'" That was to show me what kind of a person he was. Nobody else would work with him. He had to have someone. He was a bastard. He worked until he was 80-some years old.

So, there I was, setting up a household and working and dealing with my husband, who wasn't getting better. I talked him into going to school. He was smart enough, but he wouldn't take finals and never went back.

My parents were nonplussed, I think. They had not tried to stop us from going to Alaska. I'd graduated from school, and they believed I could decide where I wanted to work and who I would marry. My mother told me later she'd had to force my dad to go to the wedding ceremony.

I dealt mostly with dogs in Fairbanks. There was an enormous number of huskies with broken back legs because they fell out of pickup trucks—as many as three a week. I got good at orthopedics. People go up there and say, "I'm living in the wilderness; I want to get a husky or two or three." Then they'd throw them in the back of a pickup truck and expect them to be able to stand. They'd drive through the ice fog, and the dogs would bounce up. Some cats too.

The town was full of oilmen trying to get themselves in on the ground floor before the pipeline started. Fairbanks had become rotten.

In Alaska, everybody worked together in those winters. You learned how to handle the cold. I learned how to make parkas myself. You plugged your car in. You put in a battery heater. You used a blanket and an oil heater. It was 52 degrees *below* zero. Machinery doesn't work in that weather. The tires are hard. You'd stop and the tires would go clunk, clunk, clunk.

I got divorced in 1974; that's when it was finalized. At that time, when I first went before a judge, there was a long delay period. Secondly, the judge objected to the fact that I did not change my last name to Peter's name.

When we got divorced, my mother said, "He was too badly wounded emotionally. Emotionally complex." He was harmed. Complex PTSD. When I met him again years later, he was living on the road and in the backseat of a Saab. But his shirts were folded military crisp.

After my divorce, I spent a winter in a cabin with a guy called "Bullshit Mike" by the native people. The cabin was between the villages of Stephens and Beaver on the Yukon River, and the guy I was with was a fellow whose previous girlfriend had died out there. It was remote. Wolves, bears, foxes, and lynx. We had a sled dog team. There were also animals that wanted to eat us.

My values changed, and I started not to have things. I learned what was important.

I realized that a person needed food, water, clothing, and warmth. Also, some people and amusement. You needed something to engage you; it could even be a game of solitaire. But there are easier ways to discover that than living in a cabin in the Alaskan bush. I don't recommend anyone to do that.

When I was in the bush with the outhouse, if you went to the outhouse at 60 degrees below, the trees would be like crystal. We kept a two-inch foam pad to sit on the toilet. Fog from your mouth made ice crystals and sparkled in the air, like a Walt Disney effect. All the trees had frost on them. There were little sparkles in the air. That's how cold it was.

I came to Fairbanks to do fill-in work and a little bit of veterinary practice. I would vaccinate cats and dogs, then stay the night at the customer's house, collect the money and go back to the cabin. There were a bunch of people in the 1970s living there like that. They were hippies. A lot of back-to-the-earth people. It was not uncommon. Three or four nights a week, though, I was out in the bush cabin. I was recovering from the divorce.

Even in Fairbanks, people would have five acres of land and they cross-country skied to work. It was an alternative to being a flower child. When one of my friends talks about pop culture from the late 1970s, music and that, I don't know it. They say, "Oh, yeah, you were in Alaska in a cave under a bear." I was an earth mother.

I returned to Fairbanks after a year in the bush when I realized the guy nicknamed "Bullshit Mike" was way too weird. I lived with a friend for a while, then went back to Milwaukee and my continuing education. The latter wasn't required, but my dad suggested that I do it. I had quite a bit of veterinary equipment in Alaska. I'd bought an entire surgical kit in veterinary school and picked up other stuff over the years. My books, too, were in Alaska. But when I got back, I wasn't sure where I would work. Then someone from the Whitehorse, Yukon Territory, told me the local vet had stopped practicing. Prices were sky high in Fairbanks; you couldn't rent anything. It was a boomtown.

So, I moved to the Yukon to start my own practice.

CHAPTER FIVE

Wild in Whitehorse, Yukon Territory

To keep bears away while picking fruit alone,
recite poetry aloud.

In the summer of 1975, Whitehorse, Yukon Territory, was frontier. There was no board exam to get a license to practice medicine, so all I needed to do to start my clinic was to buy a business license.

I opened my practice in my house, so the space was half clinic and half home. Nobody minded that I was a female vet. They were happy to have a vet.

At the time, I was with a man named Michael Stackhouse, whom I'd met in Fairbanks. He was a janitor. We got married on the "marge of Lake Lebarge," which is right outside of Whitehorse, Yukon Territory, and part of Robert Service's poem "The Cremation of Sam McGee." So, I was married at another poetry-related site. Something about me and poetry, I guess.

Whitehorse in 1975 was quiet and rural and had a small downtown. A forest fire had damaged the area. You drove through big, dark sticks for miles and miles. If you went toward Dawson City, you'd see a beautiful forest.

Residents were more cautious, more conservative. It wasn't a province. There were a lot of Native Americans, and I got to know many of them.

To keep bears away when I was picking berries, I memorized poems and said them aloud when I was alone. I still remember Service's poem "The Cremation of Sam McGee." At that time, if you went to the bar in White-horse, Yukon Territory, and recited that poem, someone would buy you a drink. It was worth memorizing.

The first stanza goes:

There are strange things done in the midnight sun
By the men who moil for gold;
The Arctic trails have their secret tales
That would make your blood run cold;
The Northern Lights have seen queer sights,
But the queerest they ever did see
Was that night on the marge of Lake Lebarge
I cremated Sam McGee.

There were several other lengthy poems I memorized. I also memorized Edgar Allan Poe's "The Raven," Service's "The Ballad of Pious Pete" and Rudyard Kipling's

"The Ballad of East and West." I gathered berries, but I was not the only one out gathering berries. There were bears out gathering berries. They don't want to confront you, but they wanted to get the berries. If they heard you, they went away. I memorized long narrative poetry, so I could say these aloud without seeming like I was totally bonkers.

And I was never bothered by bears.

Michael and I were in Whitehorse for three years. I got immediately pregnant and my first daughter, Jennifer, was born in Canada in 1976. It was a rough birth. I was working right up until the baby was born, and I was exhausted and maybe had a cold, so I was coughing. I had a prolonged labor for two days. The uterus didn't expand. I was delirious. My husband didn't want me to have a C-section because he didn't want a scar. But I gave them permission.

Two days later, Michael won the five-dog race in an international dog sled competition. I walked out of the hospital with a baby and went to the awards ceremony where he won. Jennifer was 5.4 pounds. Small. I smoked when I was pregnant, but I cut back to five cigarettes a day. The low birth weight is not surprising with that.

ॐ

I handled a lot of veterinary surgery. I even created one surgical procedure that helped save a dog's paw. I sent it into the American Veterinary Journal—though I knew nothing about publication. They said, "Well, the article's clumsy, but it will work." And they wanted a lot of revision, but it wasn't clear how they wanted it revised. They damned it with faint praise.

I kept myself busy with my one-person practice in the Yukon Territory. Dogs got their paws stuck in traps and often the traps caught their front three toes, especially the middle toe. This stopped their circulation—and froze the paw. I created a system in which you save the middle toe. When they walked, their feet splayed out. I worked with the bone and the tendon to save the paw then cast it for a time. The dogs not only walked again, but they ran as normal dogs, not disabled dogs.

A few years later, I saw a surgery book with my surgery in it! I didn't know enough at the university level how someone would steal someone else's work and the level of competition. This vet didn't want me to get credit for it. But I know where that came from.

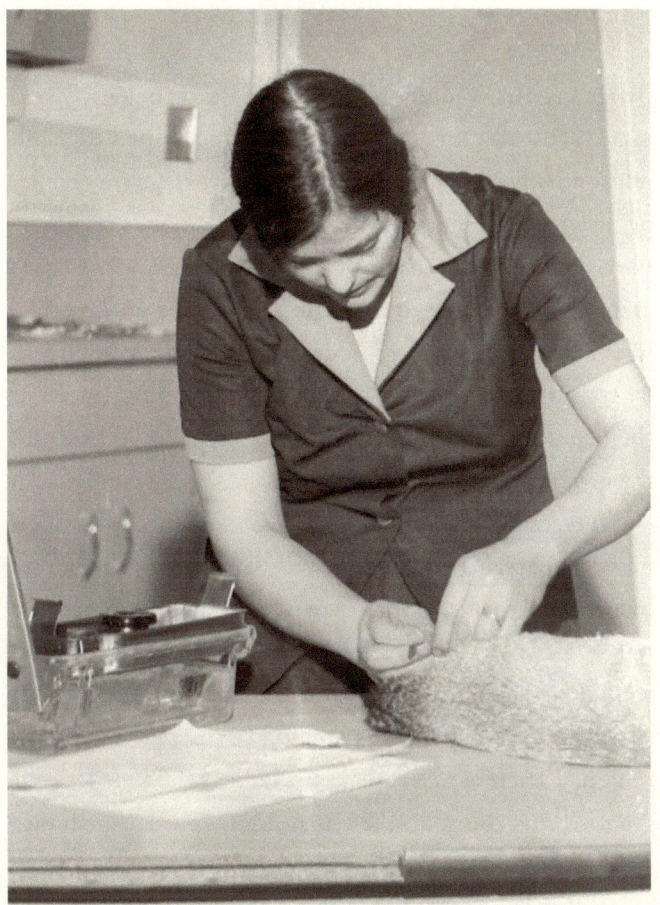

Holland handling vet work.

Being a vet in Whitehorse was wild. I was the only veterinarian for 500 miles around. My clinic helped cats and dogs, mostly, and people would send their cat to me by plane with broken legs. I often met small planes at the airport. The dogs were sent by plane, too. I did some horse castrations and helped cows. You never knew when they were coming. People got used to the snow and cold. It was up to the pilots whether to fly. They were experienced. If they couldn't tell the difference between the ice fog and the ground, they didn't fly that day.

A vet's work could be dangerous. Once, a stallion needed neutering, and no one wanted to do it. The horse's owner said to me, "Don't worry, the horse will act just fine." I gave the horse a sedative, and occasionally, you could reverse their reaction with an injection. Rarely does an animal get hyper. This stallion got hyper. The horse took off. There was a rope in his halter. The kids let go. I grabbed this thing, and it was heading toward the house with storm windows. Those storm windows were close to us! But I got in position so I could twist it and pulled it up and gave it a jerk. The horse slipped, but he was out of danger. Then the nasty owner gave me half of the pay because he thought the horse had been injured. What a jerk.

Another time was just as strange. There was a railroad that went from Whitehorse to Skagway. It was a lovely trip, all day. It stopped during lunch hour at Bennett Lake, where they had a lodge with homemade bread, hot dogs and beans and salad. That was it. Bread, hot dogs and beans and salad. Everyday. For a trainload of people. A big woman ran it.

Early one morning, I got a call from this woman at Bennett Lake who said, "My cat has broken its leg." I told her to bring it to my clinic and take the train. I said, "Put the cat in a box. It will be fine. I can fix the leg." I often told people to put the cat in a beer box which had holes and was heavy and strong.

Later, she called and said, "I'm having a hard time keeping the cat in a bag." She had been having a drink in bars at all these different stops. She was more and more slurred. She finally arrived after I closed, and she skidded up to the clinic. I had a big gravel road. She popped out of the back of a vehicle, and she had a broomstick in her hand and a box at the end of a broomstick. The cat was yowling in this box. She had the cat duct taped to the box!

The cat was in shock—and the owner was drunk. I treated the cat for shock then 24 hours later fixed its leg. She paid me half and never paid the other half. She never went back to being the cook on the rail line. Instead, she made a living sewing moccasins for tourists.

Months later, she brought another cat back in with a needle and string in its throat. It wasn't uncommon if you're sewing, and you have a needle in a pin cushion that cats would eat it. Then they wouldn't be able to close their mouths. I took care of the cat.

I also helped Whitehorse use more humane methods of euthanasia. I spent three years in Whitehorse, but my second husband, Mike, turned out to be like my first husband. He spent his time staring out the window.

When my first child, Jennifer, was born in White-horse, I overworked, I'm sure, during the pregnancy. I worked 14 hours a day and carried and lifted. Nobody else was cleaning my clinic for me. I'd get up in the morning and do all that. It was a characteristic, rural thing. The first delivery was bad. It was rough. A long labor. Forty hours later, the whole thing became static. They had to do a C-section.

During the birth, when they said to me, "We have to do a C-Section," Mike said, "Oh, no, I don't want you to mess up your beautiful belly." It's not what to say in those circumstances.

In Canada, the annual cost of healthcare was $149 for the whole year when Jennifer was born. In 1976, though, my husband wasn't interested in buying insurance. He thought it was a con game. I had to have a baby, but they wouldn't see you in Fairbanks without $1,000. So, other women waited until you went into labor and went to the ER and prayed. That was not a safe thing to do. There was no pre-natal care in Fairbanks without insurance.

We were in Whitehorse from the summer 1975 through the fall 1978. In 1978, I was pregnant with my second child and worked with a couple of vets. We still had no health insurance.

During that time, it was tough to raise your first child while working full time in Whitehorse with a depressed husband. It was really a trick. Mike was less than useful. I wasn't thinking clearly when I selected people for my life partner. Maybe he used me. Veterinarians make a good living, but not that good. Mike had gotten a homestead off Yukon farther down by the canyon, in the middle of Native land. He had to go live out there.

We moved back to Fairbanks. After our first baby was five months old, Mike spent part of the winter in a cabin. My mother came and spent some time with us. After caring for my first child alone, I wasn't going to do it with two kids. I decided to return to Milwaukee, a more civilized place, where I'd have my second baby. I had my second daughter there.

Mike was mad. He came down to Milwaukee from Fairbanks to see me. He left all my stuff up in Alaska, but he had all these big dogs because he was dog mushing. He was a hippie who played guitar; he still does, back in Fairbanks. He wanted to be supported by his wife.

My second child was born in 1979 in Milwaukee. Her name is Anna. I didn't know whether to return to Alaska or stay home. I really hadn't considered what to do while I was pregnant.

Both of my daughters turned out to be very intelligent. Jennifer lives in Portland now and works as a school principal. Anna did not go to college, but she has written books, including the popular sci-fi novel "A Long, Long Sleep."

Back then, I told Mike that he had to get a job and stop playing in the woods. He applied for several jobs. It was clear to me he didn't want to work. He would work until he was qualified for unemployment, then quit or find a way out and receive unemployment compensation. He did that maneuver three times.

In 1979, I decided not to go back to Whitehorse or Alaska, so he came down to Milwaukee after Anna was born. When I told him I wasn't going back, he was mad.

I got a part-time job then a full-time veterinary job in Green County in southwestern Wisconsin. I worked there for a couple of years. Mike came down and we made a try to stay together, but we failed miserably. He was supposed to do childcare and he couldn't do it.

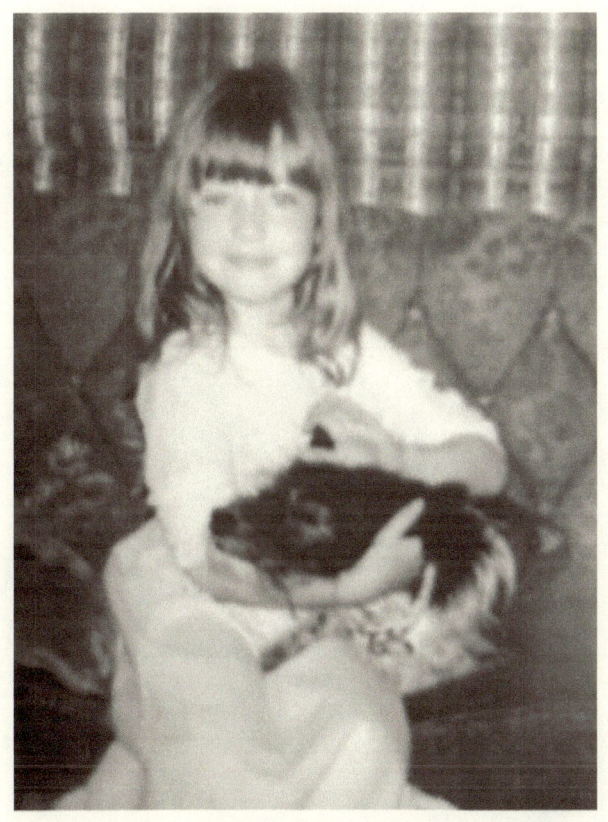

Jennifer with Ragsey.

CHAPTER SIX

Night Terrors

What keeps single moms going?
What else are we going to do?
We do what we must do.
We're scared to death that we might not live
until our children grow up.

I rented a house about 10 miles from Monroe, Wisconsin, in 1979. I worked there in a clinic with seven practitioners, six of whom were large animal practitioners.

The guys who owned the Monroe clinic didn't make it easy for anyone to buy in. It was a wide practice—they took care of cattle, and I took care of small animals.

My second marriage was falling apart, and child support for Jennifer and Anna was sparse. In 1981, Michael gave me only $1 to get clothes. A dollar doesn't buy winter coats for the kids. It was an insult. We lived at the edge of town. He came down with the dog sled. He was supposed to be looking for a part-time job, and he had depression that I didn't know about. There was a stray dog that would try to get some food from his seven dogs, and once he ran out with a gun to shoot the stray dog.

Jennifer had night terrors. She would scream at night and not be awake. She'd stop and you'd put her back down again. I would lie down next to her. I'd lie there for an hour and a half. That got old.

One evening, I went outside and saw the stray dog. He ran into the garage and sat on an old chair we had in there, crouched down on his side. His tail was wagging. He was about 12 pounds, a little thing, a cross between a beagle and a chihuahua. I reached over and he licked my fingers. This was not a vicious dog. This was a pet. I petted him and he came over to me. I brought him to the house. I went upstairs with this dog, and I curled up next to my daughter. The dog stayed there. My husband came home and shouted, "What is this dirty dog doing next to my daughter?" He woke up Jennifer and she started to cry. We washed the scruffy dog, and Jennifer cuddled up with him. The dog would lie next to Jennifer, and she never had another night's terror. We named the dog Ragsey and the dog lived with us for 11 years.

In 1982, I was about 37 years old and single—twice divorced—with two young kids. I didn't get along with the other practitioners in Monroe; we did not have the same style. I don't think they really accepted the idea that I could make decisions on my own. They were the old-style guys in a small town. When I did the first interview, they asked, "What's going to happen if you get pregnant again?"

I decided to open my own clinic in Madison, Wisconsin, and they were happy to see me go. I bought a map of the city and marked up all the zones where you could build a veterinary clinic and circled ones where there wasn't one. Then I looked for empty buildings.

Once you're a single parent—a woman with small children to care for—you almost must work for yourself. Otherwise, you're just not going to get the same flexibility. I can't imagine how other women handle it. I was so lucky in my career that I could do that.

And especially when one of your kids is disabled, you need that flexibility. You don't know when you're going to have to take off. I was lucky. We had a middle-class life. My ex-husband Mike gave me $100 a month for 10 months out of the year per child, probably one quarter of what a court ordered. I couldn't get more. He'd just say, "I don't have money this month." Financially, we were just very careful. I didn't have extra to spend. Single parents don't put money aside to raise kids.

It was a lovely place to live. I found a house on Madison's west side with a lease and an option to buy.

I knew that my second child, Anna, was autistic from day one. She wouldn't let me hold her to nurse her—I hovered over to get the nipple into her mouth. She was a different person very early on.

My first child, Jennifer, was bright, assertive, and talkative. My mother said, "Your next child is going to be more average." Anna was diagnosed with autism by a behavioral clinic at the University of Wisconsin at age six. She had lots of differences in how she interprets stuff. Lots of repetitive actions. She memorized everything.

Anna learned to read and write. She has an IQ of 135, which is a saving grace for someone with autism. People with normal IQs and autism tend to be seen as developmentally disabled. They don't adapt themselves enough to be able to express themselves for people to know what they're thinking. A lot of kids that have autism are accidentally abused early on. People expect someone to pick up their socks and they can't obey. Sometimes when things are put down, they go into a black hole in space, and they might as well not be there.

I hired people to help her after school. One woman, absolutely wonderful, worked with Anna for seven years.

It's almost impossible to get good help if you don't pay well.

Meanwhile, Anna's sister, Jennifer, thrived. She was incredibly social, relatively anxious. A ballet dancer.

I was very isolated. I didn't go on even one date. The whole idea of having another person around was too much.

What kept me going? What else was I going to do? You do what you have to do. I was scared to death that I might not live until my children grow up. This is true of everyone I talked to. No one else would take care of her. And that attention for Anna left Jennifer feeling alone. Jennifer was a good student, everyone liked her, and she was a beautiful dancer. It was hard on her. At the ballet studio, she took summer ballet and had time away from the stresses of her life. Anna's not an easy person to hang out with.

Anna wouldn't follow directions. She wouldn't come when called. If we went to a store, she would just walk off. Now, there are whole books on pervasive demand avoidance. Back in the 1980s, they didn't have anything. Autistic kids? It was like, "Give them a raisin when they're being good and hit them when they're not." There were many terrible, abusive programs for autistic children.

I got a little loan to start my veterinary practice in Madison. Years later, the guy I got the loan from came to my office. He looked at me and said, "You look so tired." But I told him about the practice and said it was going fine. I told him how I adapted. He sighed. He said, "They're closing the loan office." Then he said, "Yours is the only loan I made that worked."

Keeping my veterinary practice small and not having expectations to expand and going overboard was the way to go for me. I needed to make enough money, but I also needed the flexibility to make time. I had one, sometimes two, people working in the office. But I needed that flexibility to take care of emergencies with Anna.

Jennifer and I had some contention by the time she got into high school. I told her that I couldn't afford one of these big, expensive ballet schools. She was really ticked off and wouldn't talk to me. Years later, she said to me, "I wouldn't have been happy at one of those places." She didn't realize that at the time.

In high school, Jennifer worked and hung out with her boyfriend. She decided she would pay for school on her own, and after graduating high school, she disappeared for six months then came back and said, "I have it." She had been working.

She applied after one year off, then went to the University of Utah for ballet.

Both girls are very gifted and bright. Very bright. Both

are capable in many ways. But Jennifer has always been anxious, which takes the form of being a perfectionist. Sometimes the effort is too hard, and she freaks out. She doesn't freak out in public, only with me. When Jennifer reached her teens, she was a ballet dancer and good in school. Now, Jennifer works in education as principal of a school in Portland; Anna has written two novels, including a sci-fi book that was bought by a major publisher.

Jennifer started college the week Jerry Garcia died in August of 1995. At the time, I was driving out on Highway 80 to get her to Utah, and there were lots of VW microbuses. We ran out of gas. A guy named "Loam," who was heading to a tribute for Garcia, got us gas.

A week later, I started med school.

CHAPTER SEVEN

My Roots

*A 1950s childhood was not perfect
by any means.*

I was born March 18, 1945, in Flint, Michigan, the youngest of three children. My sister, Ellen, was born in 1940. She got her law degree after she was 40 years old because first she had gotten a PhD in 18th century literature. My brother, William, was born in 1943. He was a major executive for Weyerhaeuser, a lumber company.

My mother had a fourth child, Edmund, but he died during birth.

I was heavily influenced by my parents. My father came from practically nowhere. He was one of a family of seven from a little farm in rural central Illinois. He and my mother are buried there in a cemetery, along with his parents.

There were three boys in his family. They always said, "The family worked on the farm." My dad realized the farm wasn't going to be big enough for all of them, so he decided to get some education. He was brilliant and interested in engineering.

At the time of my birth, my dad was an executive at General Motors, which had a lot of military contracts. They were developing the Norden bombsite, a 40-pound and 2,000-piece tool that aided air troops in dropping bombs accurately. They put it together with women workers. The men they hired to supervise those women insulted the women and maybe even molested them.

Finally, they put dad in there and it stopped cold. Dad would never consider inappropriately grabbing a woman. He was raised to respect others. He even didn't like it when I was a child and learned the song about "sweet violets, sweeter than all the roses" because it had innuendo in it. He was a typical nice Irish man, engineer type, straightforward. He went all over the country to supervise the installation of Norden bombsight weapons.

My dad's family didn't know what he was doing during the war. By the time I was four in 1949, we'd moved to Milwaukee. They sent a dozen men ahead to pick a place for a General Motors plant. They had an office downtown and built a factory in Oak Creek, making AC spark plugs. They were starting to create a computer system. When I was in late grade school, they brought me down to see how they were building these big computers. Ladies sat at tables, soldering a thousand different wires.

Being from a teaching family, mom's relatives talked about education and raising children as part of their dinner table conversation. My mother would not categorize her own children. When we got our report cards, she would not compare my eldest sister to my brother or me. She would bring out my last report card and compare them to each other.

We were raised in the late 1940s and 1950s, so we were more wild kids. My parents chose a house in Fox Point, a post-World War II suburb surrounded by fields. The fields were later developed housing. But when we were there cows tethered. It was not a developed area.

My mother always had books for us. She did what you would call "enrichment" for the time. She was a science teacher, so she took us out into the fields, and we raised frogs, ducklings and turtles. And she read to us.

She picked "Wild Animals I Have Known" by Ernest Thompson Seton and eventually naturalist books written by renowned people like Liz Porter.

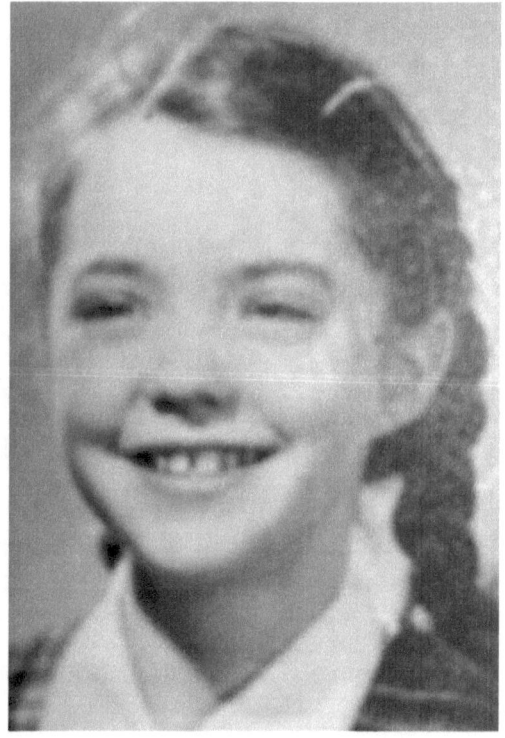

Joanne as a youth.

🐦

My parents' families came from Ireland in the early 1900s. There were two families: the McCarthys and the Hollands. They lived not too far from each other in Ireland. They went to the same church. My family thinks they had what they call "an understanding" before my father came to America, and she followed. Several cousins came to the Midwest at about the same time. Most of them settled near Bradford, Illinois, which is halfway up the state.

My father's family was Catholic and, while choosing a college, he went up to Marquette University in Milwaukee. They were nice to him. They interviewed him and the head of the school said, "Look, this is a private school. It's very expensive. What you should do is go down to the University of Illinois and get a degree there. It's a big school and you could probably work your way through. There's a Catholic student association there and you should be able to meet nice Catholic women."

And that's what he did. He worked his way through college—a freshman at age 22. It was the Depression; he was born in 1909. The family had taxes to pay, and he worked on the roads to pay the taxes off. When I was an adult, after he had a stroke, I learned more about his youth. He talked about when he was 14. He said, "I must have been shucking too much corn because my hands hurt." They had sufficient food, but not a lot of variety. Potatoes, corn, and vegetables. And what my grandma could make.

His name was Jeremiah Joseph Holland. That was how he was baptized. He was born at home. He went by Joseph all his life: J. Joseph Holland, except for his pilot license, when he worked in aerodynamics.

He graduated from the University of Illinois in engineering. He got a job with General Motors and became an executive quickly. He was a very precise man. He was a typical engineer. He didn't talk a lot. And when he did, it was all very straight and honest. His parents never said a lot.

My aunt and my father's younger sister, Dorothy, became a vice president for Kraft Corporation. Dad started the first American Society for Quality Control. They were amazing people.

My mother's father was from Oregon and her mother was from Indiana. My grandparents met in school. My grandmother was a teacher, and she taught teachers in Indiana, and my grandfather was the only male teacher at a school in Iowa, and then became superintendent of schools. He had a bad back and was always trying to find management systems for his back pain. He went to hot baths in Utah, then to the Midwest.

My grandfather's sister—there were ten children in that family—wanted him to come to Chicago. He did, but they wouldn't let him teach in Chicago because he hadn't finished his college degree. They hemmed and hawed about it. They decided to get him credit for any classes he could pass the final exam on, and he passed all of them but two. So, he went to school for a semester, and he met my grandmother in one of those classes at the University of Chicago. They were taking summer classes. Grandma was teaching classes in Indiana, and they always sent their teachers to study at a college in Chicago.

Ada Fink, my grandmother, and William Evans, my grandfather, ended up in the same Commercial Geography class. The professor was romantic. He paired them up, and they later wound up naming a son after him.

My grandmother was a Methodist; my grandfather was Catholic. That was a big deal back then. Neither family really approved.

My dad was born on Aug. 8, 1909, and Mom was born on May 13, 1913—a Friday the 13th, she always said. They dated for three years and married in 1938—in the Catholic church. They raised us Catholic; my mother used to test us on the Catechism. But they found a Milwaukee-area home where there was not an active Catholic school in that diocese, and we didn't go to Catholic school.

We camped every summer. Dad had a long vacation. These were orderly people, so one summer we would spend time at my dad's family home in rural central Illinois, then we would drive in the 1950s across to Oregon and spend a couple of weeks with my mother's family. And the final week would be at Lake of the Woods in northern Wisconsin. There was a lot of canoeing in the wilderness. He kept track of every penny that he spent by the date.

It was a "1950s childhood." Not perfect by any means. We had very little supervision, and often walked through dangerous construction sites.

As a young girl, I would always go out, sit and watch animals and insects. I'd watch the frogs come and go. I'd watch the insects and identify the plants. Oh, man, I could sit and watch for hours. My parents got me a chameleon lizard that I trained to sit on my hand. That lizard lived a long time.

Dad built a comfortable house. We were a self-contained family. We rarely had visitors. When dad had time off, we would go down to Illinois and see his family.

My parents did have a couple of big dinners when my dad started with General Motors in Milwaukee. He became head of sales, but that wasn't my dad's style. He had a drinking area in the basement. He set card tables up down there and people could drink.

In the end, GM moved him to the quality control program. People thought it was a downgrade from sales. He changed that position to a more honorable one. Then the Apollo program became huge, and he was named the director of quality control. He just kept going. He didn't express disappointment or anything that happened in life.

Mom went back to school when I was 12 to get her teaching certificate in Milwaukee. She also earned a master's degree. I was 14 when she went back to teaching. She took it as a challenge. She was a middle school teacher, and she went and worked at Peckham Junior High School, in a poor district.

She said, "We need to educate everyone."

She was very successful. She was a little old lady, but she took guns away from people. Other teachers would come to her school with these romantic ideas and leave in a year. Not her—she memorized every child's name. First, middle, and last. Any kid who misbehaved she would say, "So and so, what are you doing there?" They took it as respect. They viewed her as a grandmother and trusted her to help them.

CHAPTER EIGHT

Dyslexia Didn't Exist Then

When a teacher yells at students,
the volatility of language
blocks any understanding of what
the teacher is saying.

As a little kid, I adored animals. My older sister, Ellen, was an artist and my older brother, Bill, played sports. I chose animals as far back as I remember. The animals came to me. I played with them. They came out of the woods to hang out when I was there. I'd be in the middle of the woods, and a cat would come up to me. Or deer, squirrels, chipmunks, turkeys, and rabbits. I'd lie down, put food in my hands, and they would come and take it.

It wasn't dangerous, except once. A beagle bit me when I pulled a rabbit out of its mouth. I was 10. I didn't want the dog to eat the rabbit. I didn't want to watch carnage. I let the rabbit go. I don't know if it survived. The beagle then bit me immediately when I took the rabbit out of its mouth. I had a single bite in my arm.

I watched the animals closely. My mom also read us all these books, such as "Girl of the Limberlost" by Gene Stratton Porter, about naturalists. And right across the street from our home in suburban Milwaukee, there was a swamp, one of the last places in that area to be developed.

I went out there and sat and watched frogs and insects come and go and identified the plants. Oh, man, I could sit and watch for hours. We'd moved from Flint, Mich., to Glendale, a Milwaukee suburb, when I was four.

When I was six years old, someone asked me, "What do you want to be?" I thought about it, but I knew I wanted it to be something with animals and something powerful, and the most powerful thing with animals was to be their doctor. That's when I learned the word "veterinarian." People in medicine often decide early.

I was very shy. I was extraordinarily shy. I didn't particularly understand people. We were a self-contained family. We never had visitors. When dad had time off, we would go down to south-central Illinois and see his family. Nothing elaborate.

From kindergarten to eighth grade, I was a good student, not a great one, but I didn't feel like it. They didn't have dyslexia then. They called it "academic under-achievement." When it came to standardized tests, I did stellar. I was way ahead of everybody. But when it came to the classroom, I was behind. I had bad handwriting. I don't remember writing a full page until I was in eighth grade, when the teacher demanded it.

But I was intuitive and knowledgeable. I read at college level by the end of elementary school. In first grade, I remember a teacher trying to get me to read, and I was so startled. My teacher was a grumpy old lady who did not really like kids. Then my mom and another teacher showed me that words had shape. And phonics. Mother taught me.

My mom said this learning obstacle runs in our family. She said, "We're never good at rote learning. But we have great understanding." She had those qualities, too.

"I had similar problems," my mom told me.

I think she was dyslexic, but her parents were both educators. They worked her through it.

I became an avid reader, but I didn't like to play games, I didn't do sports, and I didn't have a lot of friends. In seventh grade, I realized that if I helped the librarian, she would let me stay there. I shelved books.

I read every animal book I could get my hands on. There was Walter Farley's "Black Stallion" series. And dog trainer Albert Payson Terhune's books about Lad the dog. Then I read books on philosophy. Then I read books on philosophy like I read "Silver Chalice" and Catholic stuff.

Once I learned that words had shapes, I began to do something they now call speed reading. If I got the gist of a word, I didn't have to know every letter. I got to read quickly, only after I got the shape right and I knew where the letters were going. That is how I could read those words. When they tested me and asked me to read, it took me longer, but I got all the answers.

I felt teachers didn't like me because they never came to my desk and talked to me about how I was doing. I was baffled by human interaction.

I walked to school. Then I turned around and walked home immediately after class ended. In school, I kept to myself. We had an ice-skating rink a half block from the house, but I wasn't there much.

I didn't start playing with kids until sixth or seventh grade. When I was 11, animals meant everything to me. I went from having a pet goldfish to a chameleon to a bird to a cat to a dog.

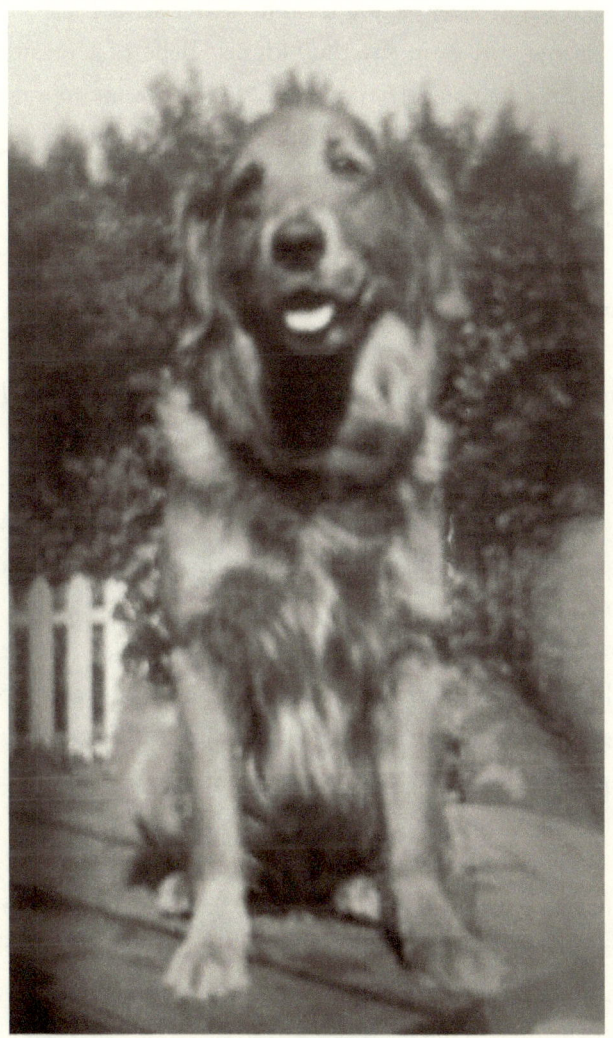

Honey Belle.

What saved me was dog training. After school, I would go home and train my dog, Honey Belle of Crossway Corner, a golden retriever. My father drove me to a dog training club. It was my dog, a CD or companion dog. Honey Belle became a state champion.

My family camped, and the dog always came along. I was massively car sick on the road; my parents would tell me to take deep breaths.

One summer, I went down to my uncle's farm in Illinois and learned even more about animals. I absolutely loved it.

I would go outside and disappear inside the barn. I would talk to the animals and hang out with them. It was wonderful. It smelled good to me, too, with all that hay and straw and manure.

My aunt, who lived in Chicago, noticed my activity when she was visiting the family farm. I changed into jeans and went outside with a bucket to feed some of the pigs, and she watched me going out there, determined and happy. She said, "Joanne, you'll retire on a farm."

My genuine care and love for animals came naturally. I have a granddaughter who is the youngest child of my oldest daughter, and she has a similar relationship with animals. It's weird. Neither one of my daughters has that, but she does.

When I was young, I knew every animal in the neighborhood. We lived at the corner of Crossway and Bell, later changed to the street named Regent. There was a man down the street, Mr. O'Connor, who had a German shepherd. He trained the dog at the football field late in the evening after work. He did a wonderful job. At age 7 or 8, I would go and sit alone and watch him. I borrowed my neighbor's cocker spaniel, Corky, and got permission to take him for walks. I saw how Mr. O'Connor trained his dog, so I taught Corky how to heel. Then I brought Corky to an obedience show.

I trained Honey Belle in obedience classes from the time she was eight weeks old. My father made an indoor/outdoor gate for the garage. Cats were in my room. Honey Belle came when she was told to come. According to hand signals, she heeled, she sat, she did a long down, she retrieved, she walked ahead, she walked to the left and she jumped over a hurdle.

I won the dog training championship with Honey Belle the summer when I was in eighth grade. I also did some teaching of dog training and working with other dogs. The club was a friendly group, Milwaukee County Dog Training.

I was 14 when Honey Belle won the state championship in the enormous Milwaukee Auditorium. But the guy who ran the dog training club, when I got the state championship, said, "Joanne, you should have been very proud up there. But you looked almost abashed at getting that award." I did not like public attention. I never got taller than 5-foot-5. They were always weighing me, and they called me Bitsy.

I had Honey Belle from the time I was nine until sixteen or seventeen, and she died when I was in high school.

I did a lot of horseback riding, too. On Saturdays and Tuesdays, I rode, and on Sundays, I went to dog training. My riding coach called us "the cavalry." He was rough. I learned to ride cavalry style, which scared the hell out of me, but I learned to follow instructions and I did well. I won ribbons there and began to work five to six hours per day.

My family bought our first TV in 1952, but it was put in the cold basement—on purpose. If I wanted to watch "Howdy Doody," I had to wrap myself up in a blanket. TV wasn't the center of our house.

I went to Nicolet High School for all four years in a Milwaukee suburb called Glendale. My sister was always a better student than me. I got a D my first semester in math, then thrashed my way through it and got a C the next semester. My mom said, "See how you're improving!" But when I took standardized tests, I answered the questions correctly. I understood the concepts. I just couldn't read the words.

During my freshman year in high school, my math teacher made each student stand on their desk. I had two math teachers who got awards for being great teachers in high school, and he was one of them. He had spent seven years in the military and taught math like he was still in it. He appealed to boys, but he seemed aggressive to me. He'd shout, "You can do this."

It worked for some people. It didn't work for me. He wanted everyone to shout, and I didn't want to shout. I didn't come from a shouting family. It inspired some people and focused them, but I didn't have trouble focusing. When he yelled at students, the volatility of his language blocked out any understanding of what he was saying.

It was an abysmal time for me. I got a D in math. The next semester, I did a little bit better. The next year, I had an older gentleman as my math teacher, and he just got up there and taught us. It sounds boring, but—bang, I learned it. He was an old-style teacher.

I didn't have trouble with chemistry or biology. I was stellar at science in general. When I learned something, I got it. I did that with math through college. But I still had such bad handwriting.

In high school, I also did art. Some teachers thought

I should study art and asked if I was sure I wanted to go into science—"I'm going to be a veterinarian," I told them.

I hung around a subset of kids who weren't happy in high school, but we went on to high achievement later. We were complex people. It took us some time. We grew up in odd ways. We—and me, in particular—didn't fit in like other kids. I don't have any nostalgia for the 1950s.

The best class I took in high school was an ecology class, and it was run by a guy who was also an artist. We went out and counted plants in a square; we banded birds; and went through swamps and looked at sedge moss. We looked at tree growth. Very, very hands on. It made me so happy.

I graduated in 1963. I was 18. I applied to veterinary schools, but I had no idea what hurdles I would face.

CHAPTER NINE

My Classmates Were Lovely

After major surgery, you need to memorize
something: take a class or learn something new.
Learn anything ... learn about all the blackberries
that grow west of the Cascades.
What will happen is your mind mends
and becomes sharper.

To apply for med school, I wrote two letters with my application about why I wanted to go. In one, I talked about my age. In the other, I wrote about why I wanted to be a doctor. "The main problem right now in medicine is access to medicine," I wrote. And I still believe that. There was no trouble for people getting access to medicine when they had sufficient money and a good job.

But the access to medicine for most people was abysmal, and I wanted to be part of trying to change that.

The letter I wrote was poignant enough that one of the people on the application board said, "Look, this is an activist. We need people who are committed to doing something about our healthcare system." That's probably what pushed me to the accepted side of the list.

When I started medical school in fall 1994, I asked a professor if he would mentor me for an elective on national healthcare. He said, "We don't have any national healthcare." I said, "I know. How about how people get national healthcare in other countries? How did the physicians act?" Everywhere they started national care, physicians fought tooth and nail against it. Doctors are a conservative group. Universal healthcare systems came from resounding pressure from ordinary people and political pressure.

That professor eventually went to Harvard and took my class idea with him.

There were two or three other students interested in helping start Physicians for a National Health Program. It was one of the first groups of that kind, which I'm proud of. I still get their newsletter.

Not everyone cheered my decision to attend medical school. My mom's first reaction to me going to med school was to shrug, "Really, dear."

I love that. She wasn't encouraging or discouraging. Later, she said, "We're very proud of you."

But she added, "We would have been proud of you had you not gone to medical school. But thank you for doing that." I have a mild regret that I didn't tell my dad I was applying for medical school. He would have been delighted. I thought it was kind of a longshot to get in, though. He got leukemia and died in 1994.

I could have gone to work for a national healthcare organization after graduation from med school, but I wanted to do patient care. I always got my greatest joy out of sitting in some little room and fixing some little problem that needed knowledge. I found it fun.

Other med students treated me well. They were students who were good at medical school, you know. Some of the older teachers were very skeptical of me. I mean, I wasn't the best student by any means. But the students were lovely. They were sweet and so hopeful; so young and delightful. We'd have discussion groups and there were all these 23- to 26-year-olds—and me. I was even older than the person teaching the class.

One year, we came back from Christmas vacation and talked about our holidays. The girl sitting next to me was 24 years old. She said, "My mother just got diagnosed with cancer." Her mom had been coughing and she had small cell carcinoma. No other student said anything. I said, "Oh my God." I took her hand, "Are you OK? *That* was your holiday?"

Everyone else was sitting there saying, "Oh, I went skiing." Nobody else seemed to know how a parent's illness might affect this student.

She didn't break down, but she said to me, "It was the worst weekend I've ever had. Everybody kept asking me about it as if I knew everything about it. I just started medical school and they're asking *me* as though I knew anything about what we're going to do."

These poor kids had no idea how to react. Next semester, they taught us how to tell patients bad news. I thought, "Let *me* tell *you!*" The students were all so sweet, but so innocent. I had so many traumas and some of them never experienced that.

Most of the other students knew I was a veterinarian. I did not say a lot about it in class. Let me tell you what doctors do not want to hear: They do not want to hear that I had done lots of surgery for 25 years. They do not want to know that their surgical technique is not as good as it should be. I had done more hours of surgery than they had dreamed of. They do not want to know that dogs and cats are really a lot like people. That was the last thing in the world they wanted to hear.

It was important to the poor fellas to have to know that they're special.

As a result, I kept quiet. I learned quickly not to give my opinion because man, oh, man did they dislike that. I rarely talked to a doctor who didn't think human medicine and veterinary medicine were extraordinarily different.

But the only difference between human medicine and animal medicine is that human medicine tends to have more rigid protocols. That's why when herbal medicine or acupuncture comes along and doesn't match one of their protocols, they have a terrible time switching over. A terrible time. They just can't do it. This has gone on for years. Then something will work, but they won't say, "I'm sorry. I was wrong." They felt superior.

During my second year of medical school, I had a shortness of breath.

When my doctor asked me about it, I said I was coughing stuff up. The joke is that when medical students take certain classes that they have symptoms of what they're learning. If you study the gastrointestinal tract for three months of classes, you may feel like you have an upset stomach. Or during the respiratory sections, everyone gets coughs, and they think they have these diseases. I dismissed my coughing. I thought it was the power of suggestion.

I went in to have my condition checked, and they did an ultrasound. This poor young woman who worked there—I could see she was scared to death during my test. She had to brace herself on the table, so her hands weren't shaking. But she saw this tumor, and she'd never seen anything like it. She watched the tumor fall from the left atrium to the left ventricle with every heartbeat. She was scared to death it was going to get caught. She went into the other room.

Without knowing what had happened, someone else in the office said to me, "You can go home, and we'll call you." But the woman who did the ultrasound took it straight to the cardiologist then they raced out to the parking lot, stopped me and put me in the hospital.

The surgeon told me what they were going to do: major surgery. He said it was the best option—the best way for me to stay alive. I said, "Look, we really don't have any choice. I do have to do it. We're going to do it." It's perfectly obvious it might not work. The tumor was huge: It was 5 centimeters by 3 centimeters by 4 centimeters. The size of a mouse.

It was a big deal. Cutting your chest is a big deal.

I was terrified. My daughters were really worried about me.

It was a big operation—and recovery took months.

But I never considered stopping med school. I was on a path. The school officials were more doubtful than I was.

I spent some time in the library researching cardiac surgery, and I came to realize that the back of your brain doesn't work well after cardiac surgery. The other thing I figured out from all that research is that if you keep on forcing your brain to learn something new that inability to think heals itself. I started believing that the thing that was making it unable to think was because you didn't have the right neuro-hormones to process the information. The only way to get it going is to learn something new. Force the DNA to make more of the complex molecules that are neurohormones.

I now tell my patients who have had all these big surgeries, "What you need to do is memorize something. Take a class. Learn something new. Learn about all the blackberries that grow west of the Cascades. What will happen is everything else will reappear. It works."

During my recovery, Anna and I watched the movie "Two Mules for Sister Sara." She absolutely loved it. That was the first time I laughed after my surgery. The movie still makes me laugh. It also reminds me of that time.

Anna was 18 at that time. She did everything for me. She cleaned the house, well, not exactly the cleanest it had been, but she was so cool. She learned how to drive, so she could drive me when I was on meds and after surgery. It was her senior year of high school.

The next spring, I was able to take some of my school loan money and paid for her to go to Europe with her French class.

The heart surgery took time to get my brain working again. I needed an extra year to complete medical school. On graduation day in August 1999, my daughters promised to come to the ceremony—if I didn't graduate from anything else ever. My mother was very ill, so we got her a condo in Madison as she became more debilitated. She wanted to live "independently." I had someone come in the morning and at night. She was "independent" for two hours. One of my daughters would see her while I was in medical school.

The last month and a half of my mom's life she was very ill, and I couldn't do anything but take care of her. I did a couple of classes, not a lot. She was 88. She had osteoporosis, all bent over. Mini strokes. Minor dementia, more over time. She couldn't swallow. On Oct. 13, 2000—Friday the 13th—she died.

Before she died, she recognized what I achieved. She was demented, not stupid.

They let me go through the graduation ceremony in August 1999, so my mother could attend, but they didn't give me my diploma until January 2000 when I finished all my credits. It was very nice of them.

Dyslexia never stopped me. It's an interesting thing. When it's combined with a kind of "giftedness," it is a different kind of thinking. I made errors of one kind or another of specifics that are very linear. It turns out image-related diagnosis is way overblown amongst dyslexics than in the average person. There are certain kinds of things that they know dyslexic people are quite good at doing now. They do very well teaching, thinking, seeing the overall picture, making decisions—and pretty good ones—based on what's likely to happen.

I was that way. I got into medical school doing that exact sort of thing: Taking the whole picture and figuring out what's the average and how would you fit that.

The University of Wisconsin medical school staff didn't know I was dyslexic. It wasn't part of any form, so I didn't see any sense in mentioning it. Sometimes I told professors if they needed to know. I talked to them casually about my age, too. "By the way, I'm 50. Let me talk to you about that," I would say. They were happy to discuss it.

I'm 79 now. Do you know how many doctors quit after 10 years? They'll work for an insurance company and evaluate people. It's a tough job. You must be strong to be willing to do it. But I diminished the number of hours to go from veterinary medicine to human medicine. And now I'm very close to the length of career that many doctors have.

CHAPTER TEN

Rough Residency

*Good surgeons
don't have time for petty stuff.*

I applied for residencies in several places. My eldest daughter, Jennifer, had moved to Oregon three years earlier, so I applied to the west coast.

After my mother died, there was nothing to keep me in Madison. So, it was off to Oregon, Washington, or northern California. I ended up in Klamath Falls, Oregon, in the south-central part of the state.

I was there for a three-year medical residency. They interviewed me in person. They were ambivalent about me everywhere I interviewed, but that was fine. Klamath Falls had several non-traditional students from other countries. It was associated with Oregon Health and Science University (OHSU). It was a rural residency. I wanted to take care of rural and poor people. I wanted to do patient care, so I went into a tiny town where they needed a doctor.

The residency started in August 2000. I had a lot of years of "stuff" and a house in Madison that I had to clear out. We packed up and packed up and packed up. I sold the Madison house and found an isolated house in Oregon. It was a chaotic period between graduating and starting my residency six months later. I had no fear of being an MD. I was sort of on track. I was moving.

I had three dogs, three cats and an autistic daughter who was 20 years old. We made three trips across the country in winter. We put stuff in storage. I found a place in Drain, Oregon. I was looking for a place that needed a doctor and a property that had to be in my cost margin after I sold the house in Madison.

My mother's father had relatives that lived in Oregon. My great grandmother had asthma and she said, "Please help me walk to the top of the hill." The boys—she had 10 children—would help her up the hill and she'd take a deep breath and say, "Now I can breathe." That was her asthma medication, and it would help my daughter later too.

I made a list on a legal pad of all the things I wanted in a house. In the Oregon valley and a lot of other places, the pollen falls in the crevices and in the valleys. You get up higher and there's less pollen. I wanted to be over 600 feet because my daughter has asthma. We found the house in April 2000, but we couldn't move in until July. We overlapped it. My daughter had an apartment of her own on this property—since I was going to be gone most of this time.

As part of the medical residency, I had to be available and near the hospital for at least one 24-hour period once a week. Klamath Falls was barely within driving distance of Drain. I had taken Anna to Klamath Falls to see if she could live there, but she choked up with asthma. She couldn't live with sage, so she was never going to live there.

So, whenever I got my 24 hours done, I'd drive back to Drain. Then I'd go back to Klamath Falls at 2 in the morning. I did a lot of nighttime driving. There wasn't a lot of time to consider whether I'd done the right thing by becoming an MD. It was hard. They want you to stay up all night, but that becomes harder when you're over 50.

In Klamath Falls, I had a little apartment for one year, then rented one room in a house. There were three-month sections during the residency doing family practice or some specialty like orthopedics or OBG-YN. I was also on call with the ER every third night.

I'd go up over the mountains then hit the road straight into the parking lot of the hospital and go to work. Most of my time was spent at the hospital in Klamath Falls.

Residencies are not intended to be pleasant. They want to break you into being a doctor. By the residency's start, I was 55. Everyone in the residency was 20 or 25 years younger. They were cute and nice. We didn't have a lot in common. We were all just busy.

I kept driving from Drain to Klamath City, which was about 90 minutes one way. Others in the residency didn't know I was doing that. They hung out with each other—but I wasn't going to go out and party. We were at different stages of our life. You sleep when you have free time.

Few people knew I had been a veterinarian, so occasionally, I would do something that would startle them. I'd be able to remove a skin tumor from someone easily. You must work your way around it underneath it. The doctor would get me started and head toward the door and I'd hold it up and say, "What do you want me to do with this thing?" They were like, "What? You're finished?"

It was difficult for some of them. Some doctors found it irritating because I had a different view of medicine than they had. After you've seen a lot of conditions in veterinary medicine for a long time, you get to the point of recognizing things. My practice in veterinary medicine was based on pattern recognition.

Doctors were basically trying to find five things that will make you have, say, high blood pressure. You list those then remove them one-by-one as a possibility. That's how they are taught to teach it. I saw patterns. Sometimes doctors were quite ambivalent about me. They thought I was jumping to conclusions. But I heard once that they said about me, "The thing about Joanne is she's always right about who should be hospitalized and who should not."

My strong opinions about patients were a bone of contention with doctors. Once, there was a 15-year-old girl in the ER in Klamath City. She was bleeding from the mouth and vomiting blood. A doctor did an exam, then, since I was the resident, I went in and checked on her. I talked with her longer than the doctor. She had had a piercing in her tongue, and it was far back. It started to bleed, and it didn't stop. The girl said she sent her friend over to buy a Big Gulp, a 24-ounce liquid, at 7-Eleven. A big thing. It was full of ice. She drank that. When she did that, the bleeding didn't stop. So, they came to the ER. She drank all this liquid. It looked like she was vomiting enormous amounts of blood.

When the esophagus breaks, you vomit blood. She was 15 years old. I knew she didn't have a serious problem. She was a skinny 15-year-old who did something stupid. I reported it to the young doctor. I said, "Well, she got a piercing. It looked like blood, but it wasn't. Then take the piercing out and put pressure on the wound until it is healed." He wanted to hospitalize her and have an upper GI done on her. She had good insurance. It covered everything. I said, "She doesn't need that!" We really differed.

The doctors called the head of my residency to lecture me. I told him, "I really didn't think she needed that." The chief resident then took me in the other room, "Jo-anne, you've got to understand." And this is my favorite sentence in the residency: He added, "This is a small poor hospital, and they need the money." I said, "Okay." They put her in the hospital and a gastroenterologist came in the next morning and looked at everything then refused to do the GI and sent her home.

The surgeons liked me. They didn't have time for petty stuff. They recognized that they could hand over a patient to close up, and I could do it and sew things up. I'd spent 20 years doing surgery half the time. Surgeons treated me more like a colleague than a resident.

There were times doctors would ask me about veterinary stuff. They were always surprised when I was right. One of my teachers had a horse and said, "The horse won't go out of heat." I said, "Change the hay. It's got some estrogen in it." Six weeks later, she came back, "We had the hay checked and it had estrogen in it." I said, "Of course." We were in the middle of a drought and that always increases estrogen.

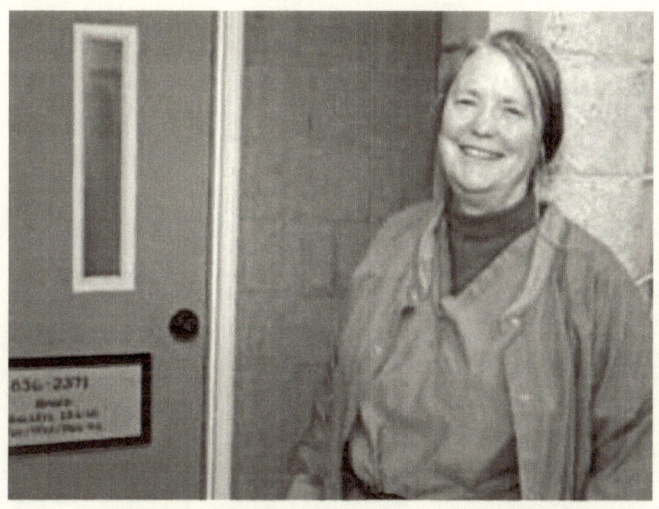

Holland in medical practice in Drain, Oregon.

CHAPTER ELEVEN

Rural Medicine Woes

We know how to fix our healthcare system,
but there is so much money involved
that people take advantage of the way
in which it is broken.

I always planned to open a rural office. That's why I picked the small city of Drain. I was looking for a place where I could easily get to Eugene or Portland to see the ballet or another performing arts show. Before my residency, I drove to all the main towns and went to the coast, checking housing and looking around. When we came through southern Oregon and passed the Drain exit, I said, "Can you imagine living in a place called Drain? Ha, ha." The next realtor showed us a house there.

There was already a doctor's office in Drain. I went in there and said, "How are you doing? Have you ever thought of having another doctor with you?" He said, "I'm planning on retiring. When can you start?" It was still my first-year residency, but I would eventually take over his practice.

I run a different kind of practice. I have a micro practice. I do it all—in particular, billing. It keeps overhead low; there are not a lot of employees.

Patients came right away when I started in 2004. Drain has 1,200 people—with 6,000 people in the whole valley. My full-time practice started just as I was about to turn 60.

Drain-area residents know each other and respect area connections, which worked well for me since my grandfather had a 125-year ranch in nearby Junction City. That impressed locals. They've been very nice to me, and I really like the people in Drain. Businesses come and go here but I'm still here, living in the community.

I see all ages, but I'm not a member of the Independent Practitioners Association. They *uninvited* me. They didn't like my prescribing habits. I would give my patients what they needed instead of sending them to a specialist when they didn't need it. The association didn't like that, but I'm too old to sacrifice my patients' need for money.

Because I'm not an association member, my Medicaid

patients are limited in number. They must go to managed care doctors. I get some who have "open cards." Medicare patients, people with private insurance, people with their own money too. That's fine. That's enough. I have many patients. I give them my private phone number.

Practicing medicine at the start was like I imagined it would be. Veterinary medicine is more flexible in some ways. Human medicine places an enormous value on *not* spending money on patients. It's amazing. If you give carte blanche, the health system can make you spend as much money as you want to—documenting stuff they should have known. I mean, a fractured leg is a fractured leg. If I know it's a fractured leg, I don't do an extra X-ray to document it. I send them to a larger facility in Slocum. I'm not maximizing how much money I can make.

And rural patients are different from urban ones. Rural patients don't see a doctor until they need it. I have patients who refuse care because they don't want to spend the money. They know it will bankrupt their family. They're not going to treat their diabetes or melanoma. They believe it won't work and worry it's overwhelmingly expensive and they'll lose their home.

It's their body. I tell them, "Look, let's see what we

can do if you let me." I might suggest the Veterans Administration to some. I tell them, "Don't deny us what we can do for you." Sometimes they do and sometimes they don't. It's up to them. I'm quite irritated by the fact that we know how to fix our healthcare system, but there is so much money involved that people take advantage of the way in which it's broken.

We came up with this healthcare system accidentally. We did not plan this. World War II came along, and we limited the change in wages. Here were these big companies: How do they get workers? They offered extra benefits instead of extra wages. They offered health care and pensions. By the end of World War II, they all had health insurance. In the 1950s, half of the country's families were covered by health insurance. There was a strong, strong feeling that this was the way to manage health care.

But after World War II, Europe was decimated. They had no such thing as healthcare. They had to come up with something and they came up with a national system in some ways. We never did that. A lot of our people were covered by employment-based health insurance. We've never had to create a system. It's a nightmare, this patchwork thing that we've got. So, we have a lot of patients, particularly in rural areas, who never had that insurance. I have patients with Social Security who get $400 or $600 per month. They get on Medicare when they're

65. They take $135 a month out of their check and the person won't get part B because they refuse to pay for it, and those people die. And they die earlier. Their hospitalization is covered, but they can't see a specialist afterward. They can't come up with the money. It's a nightmare.

That's why I went back into medicine. I had to put my money where my mouth is and that's what I'm doing right now.

CHAPTER TWELVE

Around the Clock Forever

Answer your damn phone.

I still live in the same house that I bought when I arrived in Drain in 2004. I'm still doing a life experiment. I try to live a moral life. I try to live locally, buy locally, and get as much food from my property as I can. I have 12 acres, with mini cattle and apple trees and a garden. I had a hip replacement in 2022, so I haven't been able to do much farm labor, but I still have my own eggs.

I'm a member of Gleaners in Eugene, which gathers food and hands it out to people. It's an attempt to live life in which you do things the way they ought to be done.

I'm sure I made the right decision to be an MD. Absolutely. I'm not religious, though maybe I'm a deist, but the only time I ever had 100 percent healthcare is when I had that massive heart tumor. If you were to look at that was when I had healthcare, you could say God wanted me to be an MD. There's no way I could have come up with the $145,000 to take care of my heart problem. But I was a med school student at the time, and they offered low health care insurance costs, so it was cheap. They were thinking about healthy 30-year-old men, not a late-50 something woman. If you need the hand of God showing you what to do, isn't that it?

I'm not superstitious, but it all seems to be working out as if it were planned.

My office is still open Mondays and Fridays from 3 to 6 p.m., and Tuesdays and Wednesdays all day long. On Thursdays, I sometimes work at other places.

I still do the billing myself.

Most doctors don't know what things cost. They don't know who pays what. I know all that stuff. It's amazing. Up to a third of the costs that are billed are never paid for all kinds of reasons.

One reason is that the billing system itself is not simple. You hire a biller. If you hire by the hour, they make more money if it takes longer. If you hire by the percentage that you bill out, then they only bill out the big things. I've seen them throw out little things. Hospitals hire people to do that, and they are not highly skilled. They may bill incorrectly. I asked an insurance company, "How many of these challenged bills never get paid?" And the person said, "About a third of them." They call it a denial clearance house.

My youngest daughter, Anna, lives in an apartment on my property. She has three children. If you're a parent of a disabled child, you must decide if you're all going to live together. That means coming to terms with allowing your disabled child to become an adult. They must be able to date and to make mistakes like you did.

She had a partner. They had a baby together, and her partner died of a blood clot quite suddenly after knee surgery. Their 17-year-old girl lives with us. There are two more kids, seven and nine, and Anna's current partner lives out there sometimes. Also, a handyman lives in a workshop we built out there. He takes care of the animals. I have two dogs, three cats, twenty chickens, a pony, and five little cattle.

My skills are still sharp. I don't feel like I've gotten to *not* do things. I'm walking without a cane after hip replacement surgery. I take it out to remind people not to bump into me.

I have good genes, I think. Most of what I do is give advice. I say to other elderly people, "Don't live alone." If you do a lot of living alone, it's difficult.

I knew this lovely lady who was living alone in a house of her own. But one day she couldn't get out of the bathtub. It's unwise to live alone. You should maintain your friendship patterns and make more friends. Keep doing things with people. It's tragic living alone—and rural communication is poor. I know two people who lived alone who have died in various stages of decay.

For safety, you need to have contact every day. Multi-generational families are a good way to do that.

How are human patients compared to animal patients? Humans are odd as patients. If you hurt a dog, they try to bite you. They try to get away, they snap. Human beings will say, "Thank you, doctor" when you say you're going to do something. They're extraordinarily polite. Human patients are wonderful.

My patients are also very conservative. They don't agree with my political views. They trust me, though. They know I'm going to be honest with them. I really like my patients.

In human medicine, there is more "health maintenance." We check them regularly. We're trying to keep them from getting sick. We give dogs their vaccinations but outside of that dogs don't come in until they are sick. Veterinary medicine is a little more like rural human medicine than city medicine. There's a lot of city folks going in for reassurance, "Yes, you're doing this right. It's perfectly normal." You don't get that in rural areas. I have a hard time talking my patients into getting some of their illnesses treated. I say, "We treat that, you know."

It's amazing when you think about it. I've been seeing people since 2004. Now it's 20 years. A lot of people practice medicine for 20 years and leave medicine and no one blinks an eye. People think of that as a full career. I've had two full careers now! I've been lucky to have only had diseases I could recover from.

After I've been seeing pathology for years and years and years, you get so you really can see health problems. It's uncomfortable for me. If I see someone in the supermarket and they're in the middle of congestive heart failure, I can't miss it. It's hard not to go up to them and say, "Have you seen a cardiologist?"

In a small town, I can get away with that. Everyone knows I'm a doctor. I don't know what I'd do if I didn't have the right to tell someone what they could do about some medical issue. You know sometimes people will come to me and say, "My aunt wants me to see somebody, but I've been to the ER." That's sometimes the last place you want to go if you have a complicated problem. I had a patient who said, "I've been to the ER twice and they don't know what's wrong with me." I looked at them and said, "Go back to your oncologist."

Can you imagine what it would be like if you knew someone has a bad health condition that must be treated and that you're not allowed to say anything about it? What would it be like if I stopped treating people? I don't know what I would do. I was in my early 20s treating pathology. It's been 56 years! How do I stop?

I'll say something to people about their animals too. People will bring me a pet, and I'll suggest something and won't charge them.

I feel like I've been around the clock forever. I identify as a full-time doctor. Usually when you call a doctor, and you leave a message, then a person you don't know screens through messages then decides how they'll route them: scheduling or whatever. People call me directly—and they like being able to do that. It's so much easier sometimes to just answer the damn question than to mess around with "we can't do this" or "we can't do that."

There's always the question of when to retire. I don't exactly know, but I think it will become self-apparent. I think this is now what they used to call a "retirement practice," working less than 40 hours per week. I'm mostly doing health maintenance and answering questions. I don't do a lot of surgery or procedures anymore.

Medicine has changed, especially since Covid. I do a lot of reassuring: "This is not really a conspiracy on the part of the Chinese. C'mon, now. We didn't get rid of all infectious diseases."

What's my secret for a long working life? I've been lucky in my genetics, especially when I see patients who get sick when they're young. I think I was lucky that I didn't fall into drug use in the late 1960s and early 1970s, too. I was so engaged in getting my degree to be a veterinarian that I was sort of protected. Most of my generation got sicker faster than they should have.

I learned to meditate early on too. I meditate every day. It's important. I did yoga, and I still do mild amounts of it. I write poetry. I do meditative things like embroidery and handiwork. I drank to excess a few times in college, but it got in the way of my classes, so I stopped.

But, you know, I wasn't lucky in how I picked a mate. I wasn't good at that. My daughter's autistic and I may have some of what they call autistic characteristics, but I'm not autistic.

I look at people who have long happy marriages and I don't have that. But I've had a happy relationship with my two daughters.

I don't know if it's empathy or compassion that drives me. I can feel what people are feeling and I want to make it go away.

When I was very young, animals followed me. If I was with my family and a cat was around, the cat always walked up to me. Dogs followed me. They responded to me. I don't know why. People do too for the most part. It's inherent. I think I'm a born healer. I have this overwhelming desire to make bad things go away.

Most doctors want to use big words; it makes them feel better. For me, it's really about the patients. I didn't get involved with human medicine until I realized how much people are like animals. We're just these very complex animals. My nature responds to that in a deep way.

Our culture is very strange. For a lot of my patients when I was a veterinarian, particularly upper-class people, their favorite thing in the world was their dog or their cat. That was because it was responding to them, not to their status or their importance or their position.

There are a lot of people who go into medicine who want to do this from a very early age. But it's not achievement oriented for me.

I call my clinic Pacific Gateway Medical Clinic. That's because if I call a hospital from some distance away, I can say, "This is Dr. Joanne Holland from the Pacific Gateway Medical Clinic. I'm trying to get the records for so and so." It sounds important so they'll respond. I did that from the beginning.

I've had a lot of life experiences. During my Alaska and Yukon years, I made choices based on philosophical reasons. I thought, "I won't be able to do this when I'm old and retired, so let's go."

I remember being at school with my children in Madison, Wisconsin, in the 1990s. There were a whole bunch of children and teachers on the playground. I looked up and sandhill cranes were migrating and making a big honking sound. You couldn't miss it. There was this huge flock of cranes going over their heads and the entire playground was full of children and teachers, and nobody looked up. I said to a teacher, "Sandhill cranes!" She said passively, "Oh." I never miss something like that in nature. It's an affinity.

When I was doing my medical residency in Klamath

Falls, I left home at 2 a.m. to get to the hospital. I'd drive past a little fence along my route. And there was a herd of elk, about twenty of them. The elk would come out and jump over the fence one at a time. It was just like how they show counting sheep to make you sleep.

What a wonderful thing: Animals show up for me.

Poetry by
Dr. Joanne Holland

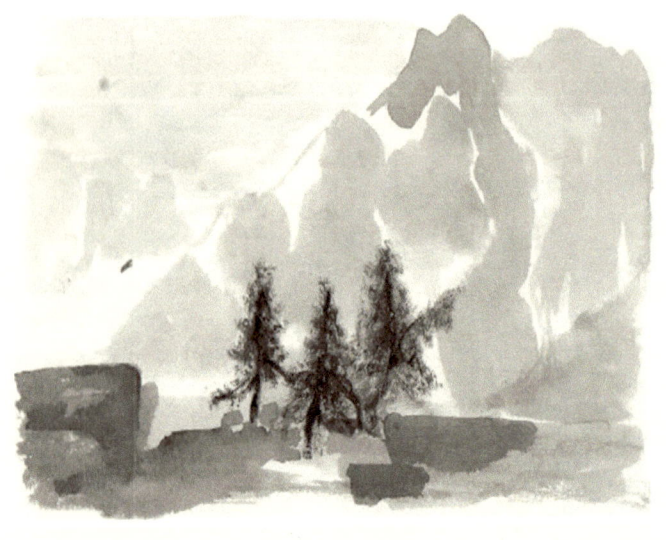

by Joanne Holland

Yukon

We caught it when we took the time
To wait the winter out.
The forty-mile distant mountain
Roared a warning shout.

The wind would rise; the river's low
Would peak and break a hole
The gunshot break would crack like
Pressure sometimes snaps a soul.
The river's lead would open and
The water hiss through snow
And there it sat and laid a trap
Of deadly overflow.

I shared the winter river sound
With someone close to me.
Saw the power of the weather
Over water's harmony
I watched the cracks and leads
Within my own integrity
And saw my weathered nature mar
Love's opportunity

Jenny

Jenny wants bright flowers of many colors.
She told me this morning
"Let me come, let me come …
Okay, then you buy them:
Be certain they have lots of colors
So the yellow sun's blood
Can help them to grow."

I went out and bought her garden.
A coat of many colors.

Anna

Anna's new, but quickly grew
Mobilized with legs alive;
They don't relate
They motivate
Not quite straight
Legs over there with arms elsewhere;
Hugs strenuous, peace tenuous.
Loves stands on laps, then lands.

Civilization Fog

The man on the river ice
Whose corpse they found in the morning
Was drunk and lost in the fog
When he turned away from the town
And strayed behind the ice floes,
They said.

A Book Came in the Mail Today

Edited by several people
Written by dozens more
Who spent many hours
Making it right.

My book's chapters have convoluted information
They interdigitate;
Their maze a sturdy mesh
To hold my mind.

The intricate systematic
Distortion of reality
Is close to right

I stretch the binding,
Turn the pages,
Caress the chapters.
I am in love.

About the Authors

Dr. Joanne Holland, DVD and MD, spent nearly 40 years as a veterinarian in isolated spots in Alaska and Canada before starting her own practice in Madison, Wisconsin. At age 54, she opted to enter medical school. She opened a one-person medical clinic at 59 in tiny Drain, Oregon, in 2004. She still works there. Holland has two daughters and lives on a small farm in Oregon.

Tom Alesia wrote the 2022 baseball bestseller *Beauty at Short* about obscure Hall of Famer Dave Bancroft. Winner of the National Music Journalism Award, he spent three decades as a newspaper features writer. He lives in Madison, Wisconsin.